Discover

Neurochemistry

Discover

Neurochemistry

Become Happier, More Confident & Creative

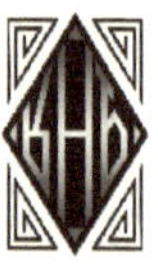

by Neuro Geeks

DISCOVER NEUROCHEMISTRY
BECOME HAPPIER, MORE CONFIDENT & CREATIVE
BY NEURO GREEKS

***

***

Paperback ISBN: 9798375940786

ePub ISBN: 979-8-2151728-6-5

***

Written by Neuro Geeks

Published by Royal Hawaiian Press

Cover art by Tyrone Roshantha

Publishing Assistance by Dorota Reszke

***

For more works by this author, please visit:

www.royalhawaiianpress.com

***

Table of Contents

Self-Test to Find What Works for You

Timothy Noakes, a famous Ph.D. in exercise science, likes to say that 50 percent of what we know is wrong. The problem is that we do not know which 50 percent that is. That is why we self-test all the scientific studies in the world means nothing to you if it doesn't help you. That is why I want you to approach this book as a hobby scientist.

The only subject in your studies is your success is when you feel better.

Never mind. Randomized double blind placebo-controlled trials. Your task is to find what works for you. If you get the placebo effect and you feel amazing Why not. When you do self-testing make sure that you do the simplest experiments to make progress. You test one variable at a time, and you keep other variables relatively constant while testing.

You will also benefit from writing a short log of tests including your hypothesis how you will measure success and your results. Jeff Sutherland writes in his book scrum that it is a fairly known rule in medicine for patients to report their perceived improvement in a symptom. It has been more than a 65 percent improvement. It's difficult to notice small improvements to keep this in mind while testing. Enjoy the process.

The Feeling of Dopamine

Imagine being able to get more creative whenever you need to do you want to be able to consistently get into more confident States. Or maybe you just want to feel better is all within your reach. You just need to understand how to stimulate the release of dopamine. Studies show that dopamine makes us more confident dopamine also plays a large role in creativity.

This is partly because it boosts your brain's ability to recognize patterns. It also reduces self-criticism. We also know that higher levels of dopamine in the brain generally enhance mood and increase body movement and that release of the neurotransmitter dopamine helps to regulate the feelings of pleasure like euphoria and satisfaction.

Do not mind makes you enjoy whatever you're doing. It is the wonderful feeling of the delicious dinner. It is the good feeling of completing a task and it is the exciting feeling. Then you go. You just set for of dopamine release is probably the easiest to stimulate out of all the most important feel-good neurotransmitters. You can stimulate release of Dark man within seconds.

If you understand what it takes some of the ways you can predictably stimulate releases dog men are setting goals. Measuring your results giving yourself rewards and also setting yourself up for unexpected rewards. Taking risks exploring meditation cold showers and getting them skosh music and food. We will cover all these and this section of the book.

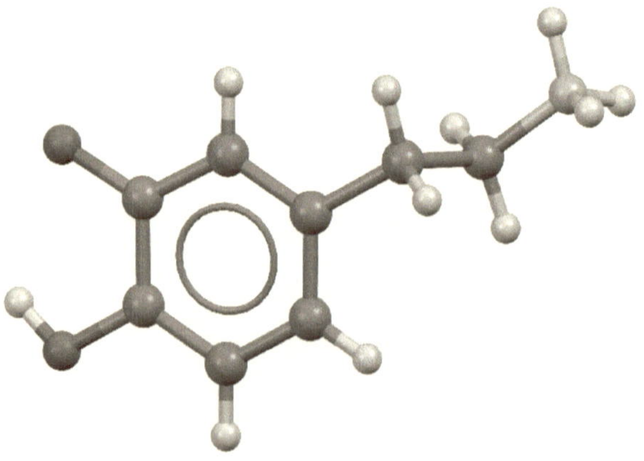

The Feeling of Low Dopamine Levels

The other side of the coin is having too little dopamine. What happens when you're not stimulating enough of this confidence and happiness boosting chemical not getting enough dopamine will lead to an imbalance that will make you depressed in the long run.

Boredom apathy chronic fatigue and even Restless Legs are in store for you if you do not build your life to supply you with dopamine unstable dopamine levels are also implicated in bipolar syndrome obsessive compulsive disorder. M.S.

Are you having difficulty concentrating low dopamine might just be the reason people with attention disorders seem to have lower dopamine levels and seek stimulus to get rid of unpleasant feelings. Do you lack motivation in your life. If we are anything like mice dopamine is probably the reason in this study, they looked at the mice that were severely lacking in dopamine even though they had constant access to food.

They couldn't find the motivation to eat. The mice died of starvation before four weeks of age. They couldn't be saved however by giving them don't mind stimulating drugs without Dopamine you won't find the motivation to go out into the world and do amazing things. You won't even get to the fridge Dopamine is also tightly linked to addiction.

It has been called the master molecule of addiction when a neurotransmitter like dopamine streams over a synopsis you hardwire certain circuits in your brain. These are specifically related to thoughts memories and circuits that motivate behavior.

Notice that Pokémon hardwired circuits are linked to motivating behavior your habits and addictions have been hardwired by dopamine. If you want to make new habits that are stronger than your bad old ones, you need to use document to your advantage. After this section you will know many ways to make dog men work for you. We start with rewards.

Boost Dopamine with Rewards

Dopamine release is strongly tied to getting rewards both expected and unexpected. Rewards cause the release of dopamine when you get an unexpected reward or an unexpectedly good one doesn't mean rewires your brain is specifically the worst part that is associated with values and goals. It also requires that part of your brain where automatic action and thinking is produced this is to steer you in the direction of past behavior patterns. This has some important implications. First of all, you can use this to your advantage by rewarding yourself when you want to create a habit or something.

For example, you can indulge in some dopamine stimulating foods when you do something important. Preferably it should be healthy foods like dark chocolate or green tea which both stimulate dopamine. The task can also become a reward in itself. You get closer to finishing you get better. You get a good conscience. You show yourself that you are a doer. All these things are rewards which stimulate documentaries.

This is a good way to turn a task into a habit by just doing Secondly it shows the importance of taking action and entering uncertain territory. If you want the high chance of getting unexpected rewards which are the most pleasurable ones, you have to take action you have to be able to handle some uncertainty. If you always do the same things never take any chances. You won't get many unexpected rewards.

It is the unexpected rewards that give you the largest releases of dopamine. It is also important to understand the darker implications of how unexpected rewards trigger dopamine release. You have probably checked your Facebook many times looking for notifications. Those red numbers that notifiers of messages friend requests and other notifications are both expected and unexpected rewards.

You get especially large dopamine releases, and those numbers are high since you get so many of these dopamine releases and some of them are quite powerful. It is easy to develop a strong habit of checking your Facebook. Some people can waste hours every day by checking their Facebook repeatedly this type of largely mindless behavior can occur in many contexts. I am not an exception. I constantly work in rewiring these habits because they can diminish my life satisfaction.

After this book you will understand better how to combat Facebook addiction and other similar addictions. Start right now by taking action on your goals or dreams. Go into the unknown by taking action reward yourself for starting and working some set amount of time. Notice the good feeling you get when you start noticing when you finish a paragraph or some other part of the project.

Notice the pleasurable feeling you get when you are near to completion and when you're completely finished wait for the feeling of an unexpected reward. It might be finding a new piece of knowledge you can use or maybe someone giving you praise for your work. Any good feeling when something occurs that you couldn't have expected. If you regularly do this and you're mindful of how you feel when you get rewards you will soon understand yourself and your actions at a much deeper level.

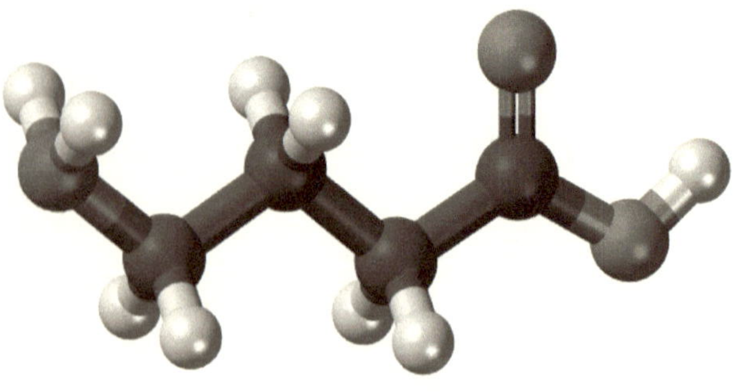

Boost Dopamine by Setting Goals

Dopamine is very important for a goal directed behavior. You can predictively get those mean by setting goals both long term and short term the main areas with set goals in our health wealth and relationships. It is advisable to set goals in all these areas because together they affect all the feel-good neurotransmitters you can set short term goals to get don't mean say need to finish a project by Friday. That is to say that's a 2:59 go through what you want to achieve today to get you closer to finishing the project.

You get a small dopamine boost just by formulating the goals and your brain starts working better. You also get a small don't mean boost from each completed task. Say you want to look more fit you can then set goals for what you want to weigh. Visualize how you want to look and set specific goals for your strength and endurance.

To take it further you can get a set number of hours of a set number of days to reach those goals. Planning it visualizing it doing it reaching both long term and short-term goals will give you recurring dopamine, but you will also get extra dopamine from all the unexpected rewards.

You feel good you get stronger. People tell you how good you look and the pain in your lower back fades away. Maybe your goal is to improve relationships with relatives and family.

You can for example aim to have 10-to-30-minute conversation with a relative or someone in your family every day or every week set aside the time to pick up the phone. You can also set goals for how you want to behave and the conversations you want to listen more than speak or get better at asking questions. Giving compliments start off by thinking about what is most important to you.

Write down one area of your life in which you would like to improve set a goal for goals. What you want to achieve the coming year and the coming week in this area now make plans for what you can do today to take a step closer to your goals. Make it something that is relatively easy to do then go through with it. Write down your goals your plans and your actions and update regularly.

You will get a don't mean boost when you've articulated your goals because you can see the promise of some reward. You will also get a Doberman boost when you've completed the tasks setting 1 to 3 goals for what you want to achieve every day. It's not only powerful and easy way to feel good but it will also result in dramatic improvements in your quality of life.

Make it a priority to complete those tasks. First thing every day cognitive neuroscience has shown us that we have a limited amount of will power and that we spend it during our day spend it wisely and early willpower also grows with. Like when we exercise our muscles. You refill your willpower during sleep. You can also partially refill by eating and drinking healthy during the day.

Boost Dopamine with Results Measurement

What we measure it improves. This is because when you measure your progress you get small victories along the way. These victories are like unexpected rewards and lead the release of dopamine that don't mean release makes you want to improve even more so that you can get more dopamine. Make your goals measurable and write down what you have done to move towards them.

Measuring your progress also gives you another benefit. We humans react stronger to loosing something in the gaining this especially applies when we have improved it and seen that you are capable of more. If you measure your results, you get poorer result than last time. This is a strong motivation for increasing your efforts but don't be too hard on yourself. You only get Dogmen if you actually view your victories as real victories. Give yourself a high five and mentally celebrate your small victories. That pleasure you feel in the moment is often called Donek pleasure.

This study advocates actually measuring your level of happiness throughout the day. The researchers' criminal buck and Ber ridge upright that supporting a hedonic approach. It has been suggested that the best measure of subjective well-being may be simply to ask people how they don't feel right now.

Again, and again so as the track their hedonic accumulation of daily life these repeated self-reports of the Donek States could also be used to identify more stable neurobiological hedonic brain traits that expose particular individuals toward happiness measuring your own happiness throughout the day to help you discover what makes you happy.

It can also lead to more long-term happiness which is related to the memory of a life well lived.

Boost Dopamine by Taking Risks

You can stimulate dopamine release by taking risks. This is because dopamine helps you react to important changes in your environment. Dopamine helps us survive when we take risks increases your focus when you need it you pay more attention you process information faster. You're more creative and your muscle timing improves I think right.

This study dopamine support brain systems are engaged in motivational sailings including orienting to detect potentially important events cognitive processing chews response and to remember its consequences and motivation to persist in pursuit of an optimal outcome. The risk doesn't have to be physical to stimulate Dohrmann release. You can be a social risk like saying hi to a coworker at the coffee machine or it can be created a risk. It takes courage.

Let go of perfectionism and be creative. That risk taking in itself stimulates though. And we also get it from the reward of surviving saying hi to a stranger could spell doom for your DNA. Tens of thousands of years ago. Nowadays you only risk having an awkward conversation about what your job description is. The potential gain is huge.

On the other hand, the guy at the coffee machine might be a door opener for a world of opportunities. Risk taking behavior is important in our modern life. It generates possibilities and documentaries. It only has to feel like a risk though for some people this could be talking in front of 5000 people. For others it might be going to the store. You have to identify what risks you need to take then you take at least one risk every day.

Boost Dopamine with Exploration

We are hardwired for exploration. We get a dopamine release every time we explore dopamine gives you that desire to investigate the world and make meaning of your surroundings. As de Young writes in this paper the general function of government is to promote exploration by facilitating engagement with cues of specific reward and cues of the reward value of information. And uncertainty is an innate incentive reward as well as an innate threat.

This means that exploration is not only encouraged by men but also the exploration stimulates release of the men. This is because the document is stimulated both by risk taking and from getting rewards. This knowledge has broad implications for how to live life if you want to stimulate dopamine he can for example, try a new route to and from work. He can step onto a different path when in nature he can try a new bar.

You can also explore inside the mind creative exploration can be a highly stimulating task with many unexpected rewards. Read new books about psychology and human nature and explore other points of view. Do some exploration every day. It doesn't have to be a big thing. Routines and habits are incredibly important but if you never shake things up your life can go stale and lifeless. Meaning low don't mean levels.

Boost Dopamine with Meditation

Thanks to science we understand more and more by meditation is so good for us. This study found something surprising. Meditation can increase your dopamine levels dopamine might be one of the reasons why meditation is such an incredibly effective treatment for depression.

There are many ways of meditating or Google could search quickly give you advice from some of the most respected meditation practitioners. The book eight minutes meditation gives you a quick introduction to eight the most popular methods of meditation. If you want to go more in depth, I can recommend the book

The Three Pillars of Zen. The quick and easy answer is that you focus on your breath and let go of the thoughts that arise. If you have never done any meditation, I can recommend these easy exercises to start sit in a straight-backed chair with both feet planted on the ground.

Set your time for as many minutes as you wish to meditate. I recommend minimum four minutes and a maximum of 30 minutes for each session. Take a deep breath through your nose and down deep into your stomach. Let both the inhalation and the exhalation last for three to four seconds. Stop for one second in between feel and focus on the air rushing over your nostrils. Take three of these long breaths and your breathing fall into natural rhythm.

Every time you become aware of the thought let it go and go back to focusing on your nostrils. When you start relaxing and your breathing slows down it becomes more difficult to notice the air rushing over your nostrils. This forces you into deeper focus keep doing this until the alarm sounds realize that you're always successful when meditating trying to success. We will revisit meditation when it is time to boost the other neurotransmitters.

Boost Dopamine with Cold Showers

The research paper human physiological responses to immersion into water of different temperatures they found that cold water immersion increased dopamine levels by 250 percent. They tested the subjects in 30 to 20 and 14 degrees Celsius. But there was no significant change in the cases of 30 to 20 degrees Celsius that data supported them thesis that responses induced by cold are mainly due to increased activity of the Sympathetic Nervous System.

This means that you can increase your dog levels by taking short cold showers. 14 degrees Celsius is a good choice of temperature based on this research you can turn up the heat towards the end of the shower to get comfortable again.

Boost Dopamine with Massages

Do you ever wonder why getting a massage feels so good. In this paper called cortisol decreases and serotonin and Outman increase following massage therapy. They found that in studies on massage therapy in which the activating neurotransmitter serotonin dopamine were assailed in urine an average increase of twenty eight percent was noted for serotonin and an average increase of thirty one percent was noted for dopamine.

They also found an average decrease in the stress hormone cortisol of 31 percent. In addition, you get several other benefits massages like increased muscle mobility and improved sleep think through who might be willing to give sources and do. I'll scratch your back if you scratch mine if they need some persuasion. You can slap this research on the table.

Boost Dopamine with Music

Music it can stimulate intense feelings of euphoria and satisfaction. And part of the reason for this is that it stimulates dopamine release. This has been scientifically proven. We have made archaeological discoveries of flutes made 40000 years ago.

Music seems to be one of the most ancient human cognitive traits in the paper from perception to pleasure music and it's neural substrates. The researchers propose that pleasure in music arises from interactions between cortical loops that enable predictions and expect in the seas to emerge from sound patterns and subcortical systems responsible for reward and evaluation.

The researchers in the above-mentioned paper compared dopamine release in response to pleasurable versus neutral music and confirm that strong emotional responses to music lead the dopamine release and the muscle limbic striatum which can help explain why music is considered rewarding. When we listen to music, we continually make small predictions for what comes next.

When our predictions are correct this is like an unexpected reward which stimulated Stoppelman Millie's fulfillment of prediction. These two Dopamine lives in the striatum with a greater response associated with better-than-expected reward there's an interesting consequence of this.

Music, you listen to a lot is not as effective for stimulating Dodman you're so familiar with the music that predicting correctly is no longer an unexpected reward. If the music is completely new to you on the other hand you don't know what to predict. Often you have to listen to a song a few times to really appreciate its beauty.

Forget the Dopamine least that gives you the chills to get the most dopamine out of music. You can rotate your playlist so that the music doesn't become too familiar also have some patients with new music might take five or 10 listening's to start up. The prediction reward mechanism.

Boost Dopamine with Food

Nutrition is a key factor for all the neurotransmitters the production of all those chemicals to make your smile widen takes a lot of energy from the nutrient's protein carbohydrates and fats. These other macronutrients.

It is also important to get large amounts of micronutrients or minerals vitamins and antioxidants. The macronutrients supply the energy or calories as well as building material for neurotransmitters micronutrients on the other hand are only building materials and contain no calories. They're the stuff that keeps you healthy and happy.

You want to maximize the number of micronutrients per calorie in your diet. And optimal eating strategy then has to include low caloric, and micronutrient dense foods like for example leafy green vegetables collards and root vegetables. A good rule is to focus on eating lots of vegetables with strong colors like green and red.

For now, we're only going into what you can eat to stimulate dopamine. You can stimulate dopamine release by something as simple as drinking tea lacking green tea contains an amino acid called L C and in l. The Indian has been shown to increase dopamine levels. In addition, you get loads of antioxidants. You might also find it highly enjoyable. I recommend steeping tea for no more than two minutes as it quickly goes better. Another fantastic drink is coffee increases your levels of Doberman. It also increases the number of dopamine receptors.

Coffee also seems to be neuro protective. It protects the dopaminergic system from neurotoxins it protects your dopamine and your Duck man receptors. Next up is Cookman this health and Hansin compound is found in the tasty spice turmeric which I personally put in almost all my food turmeric increases the level of dopamine among other things.

A trick here is the concealment together with pint Berean which is found in black pepper pre-print enhances Bayou availability of curcumin. The next drink is magnesium this study found that magnesium had anti-depressant the facts because of its stimulating effect don't mean among other things. One way to get additional magnesium in your died is the popular nutritional supplements Salomé STROMAE contains magnesium sink vitamin B6.

If you live in the higher latitudes like in Canada, Russia or Scandinavia where even a bit further south or if you spend most of the day, inside consider buying vitamin D supplements vitamin D is important in the production of dopamine and serotonin our mood has been shown significantly drop in the winter due to lack of vitamin D research and vitamin D supplementation has shown the sweet spot to be about 2000 international units a day which is the equivalent of 50 micrograms.

This is very far from the level of which vitamin D might become toxic and have been shown to be the dose that increases lifespan the most according to this study maybe the most important thing you can do for yourself is to quit eating sugar gives you a dog inspired together with some opioids. Sugar makes it feel good. For a few seconds or minutes when you eat sugar your body responds with a strong insulin response to bring down your blood sugar levels. This is to avoid brain damage among other things.

This results in very low blood sugar levels after a short while your dopamine production is dependent on having a steady supply of energy. So, when your blood sugar drops so does your dopamine your brain is unable to function properly because your boatman levels are unstable when you eat sugar unstable levels of Dopamine are strongly tied to bipolar syndrome obsessive compulsive disorders and addictive behavior. Sugar is highly addictive. It triggers the same reward part of your brain as cocaine.

This is some of the reason why some of you hearing this right now are coming up with reasons for why you can continue with sugar, and it doesn't help that whenever you try to quit eating sugar you get withdrawal symptoms.

It can take weeks to become completely free of this addiction.

There are so many reasons to cut out sugar. But this is outside the scope of this book. You need to decide what to eat to avoid blood sugars bias followed by low blood sugar. The short answer is to stay away from sugar as much as you can and try to only consume sugar while training sugar has what we call a high glycemic index meaning that the glucose is released into your bloodstream very rapidly a low glycemic index.

On the other hand, means something good cause is steadily released into your bloodstream of a long time period. This is good because you get stable levels of insulin and therefore the levels of dopamine and serotonin all the way to the next meal. One trick you can use is to replace all sugar you use in your cooking and baking with palliating nose. This is a carbohydrate that releases glucose into your bloodstream much slower than regular sugar.

The nose has been used in Japan since 1985. It's a sweet and regular sugar but it's better for you. Eat as much Whole Foods as possible. A good rule is to try to only things that your grandmother would recognize as food. Of course, in a globalized world that might get increasingly difficult as your grandmother probably doesn't know what a dairy and food is for example.

The point is they fill your fridge with Whole Foods and stay away from processed food as much as possible. Keep the low glycemic index carbohydrates because then glucose is gradually released in the bloodstream. This gives you a stable insulin level and optimum levels. If you're wondering if a food item has a low glycemic index. Google knows. But most of the time your intuition is probably true.

By five to 10 items of Whole Foods today and stay away from sugar if the craving for sugar is really strong by some sweet fruits like dates or pineapple recommended food items including broccoli cauliflower spinach kale sweet potato and beets search for recipes containing these food items and make them a part of your food habits also bison green tea steeped in warm water for about two minutes. Next up are the endorphins.

The Feeling of Serotonin

Serotonin or five hydroxy tryptamine is the calm and certain feeling that your needs will be met with high serotonin levels. You are completely content. Everything is as it should be. There is the feeling of being respected and looked up to that people come to you for guidance and want your acceptance. It has been called a social molecule and it is strongly tied to hierarchy.

We have higher levels of serotonin. You are and you feel more socially dominant. You enter a calm yet focused state you're more laid back and you enjoy social situations more. Your body is dependent on serotonin. It regulates many physiological functions like your hormone production your sleep cycle motor control immune system intake of food and energy bonds just to name a few serotonins is also important in higher brain functions.

It plays a large role in learning through its effects on synoptic plasticity or the process of brain change and neuro Genesis the creation of new brain cells. Higher serotonin levels can also increase your cognitive flexibility and make you more open to new experiences. Openness to new experiences puts you into the path of unexpected rewards which gives you dopamine boosts when your serotonin levels are elevated. A space opens up inside you.

You relax and start looking outwards becoming more extroverted. You know your needs will be met. You start looking to satisfying other people's needs. Serotonin has been shown in numerous studies to affect how we behave in relation to others pro-social and affiliates of behaviors are associated with a well-functioning serotonergic system.

Antisocial and aggressive behavior on the other hand is associated with a dysfunctional started to emerge IC system the highest serotonin densities are found in those areas of the brain that are associated with social cognition and decision making one study looked at the effects of selective certain re-uptake inhibitor see telegram on moral judgment and behavior like the authors of the study States. We show that the neurotransmitter serotonin directly alters both moral judgment and behavior through increasing subject's aversion to personally harming others.

How much the participants of the study changed in response to elevated serotonin levels was influenced by their personality's individuals high in trait empathy so stronger effects of a moral judgment and behavior than individuals. Low trait empathy together these findings provide evidence that serotonin could promote pro-social behavior by enhancing harm aversion, a pro-social sentiment that directly affects both moral judgment and moral behavior. Serotonin makes you feel better improves your social skills and promotes peaceful and cooperative behavior.

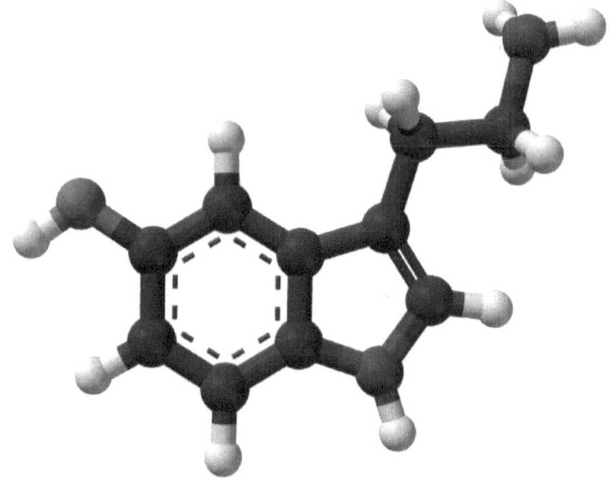

The Feeling of Low Serotonin

We commonly known serotonin from SSRI antidepressants like Prozac into teleprinter some depressing statistics tells us that then few years from 1999 to 2012 the percentage of Americans on SSRI antidepressants increased from about 7 percent to 13 percent. Depression is associated with persistent feelings of sadness anxiety pessimism irritability guilt worthlessness and helplessness you feel empty and have no interest in hobbies and activities.

Your energy levels are low. It's difficult to concentrate remember and make decisions. You have problems with sleep you get unexplained changes in appetite and weight. There are physical aches and pains that are difficult to explain, and you might even have thoughts of suicide. Not everyone who is depressed have all the symptoms above, but they tend to go hand in hand.

A low serotonin level is in many cases the leading cause of depression is also associated with a range of physical symptoms like this statin the study serotonin may be associated with physical health as well as mood in otherwise healthy individuals or low prolactin response to the serotonin releasing drug and floormen was associated with metabolic syndrome a risk factor for heart disease suggesting that low serotonin may predispose healthy individuals to sub optimal physical as well as mental functioning.

Low serotonin levels are also implicated in rheumatoid arthritis and inflammation of the gut. Low serotonin is also correlated with an inability to regulate emotions and impulsive aggression. Like the state in this study 20 separate studies found a low level of serotonin significantly contribute to aggressive behaviors regardless of type of crime and mental health problems.

A dysfunctional serotonergic system can also cause problems in the dopamine system creating further problems with the serotonin system can make life miserable. Thankfully we know many ways to improve our serotonin levels.

Boost Serotonin with Light

Have you noticed how your mood changes during the seasons maybe your mood slowly worsens from late fall until the end of winter. Then when spring sets in and especially when you have the first day of warm sunny weather your smile makes a big comeback.

Or maybe you feel a difference in your mood on rainy days and warm sunny days. There is some exciting research being done which shows that we can increase serotonin production with bright light. Light therapy is increasingly being used as a treatment for seasonal depression.

We know that we have lower levels of serotonin during winter than during summer and the antidepressant effect of bright light is likely due to its stimulating effect on serotonin production. It seems though that bright light can also work. Other times of the year like the authors of this study States bright light is of course a standard treatment for seasonal depression. But a few studies also suggest that is an effective treatment for non-seasonal depression.

In the paper light treatment of mood disorders. They found that bright light yields the best effect while dim light does not seem to be effective. They also found that light therapy gives the best results when done in the morning. They say that exposure to morning plus evening light provided no benefit over morning light alone.

Light treatment in the morning can also help you fall asleep in the evening. Evening subjective sleepiness improves with morning light. Even a short 15-minute exposure in patients with winter depression light treatment works best with whole spectrum lights. White light works better than both blue and red lights. U.V. light is not required to get a response. The best results come from light treatment with an intensity of two thousand five hundred to ten thousand Lochs of whole spectrum length.

Some examples of light intensity include a full moon on a clear nine point twenty-seven to one Loch's living room lights 50 Lux Bowfin's lighting 300 to 500 lux full daylight 10000 to 25000 Lux and direct sunlight 32000 to one hundred thousand lux. It is also advisable to do more than an hour every morning most lambs used for light treatment can stand on your kitchen table while you eat breakfast.

We can put it beside your desk while you work. It doesn't have to be an hour, or you lose, and it will improve the quality of the rest of your day. You might wonder if light treatment works for you if you're spending in excess of one hour in the sun a day with little clothing and the sun is high in the sky you probably won't get much benefit.

But we do know some indicators that light treatment will work for you. It is especially effective in winter people with seasonal mood disorders like the state in this paper seasonal affective disorder patients in particular are responsive light treatment carbohydrate craving and hypersomnia are predictors of response.

So if it is winter you feel like crap you crave carbohydrates and you need a lot of sleep. It might not be a bad idea to invest in a lamp with both of these qualities. Full spectrum lights and light intensity of 2500 to 10000 lux.

Boost Serotonin with Sunlight

This is the first day of 2068 with sunny weather and temperatures over 5 degrees Celsius Hardenberg in. I just spent two mood enhancing hours on a park bench drinking coffee and reading the story of the human body. Now I feel more energetic happy and eager.

Some light always seems to have this effect on me, and I've always been a self-proclaimed sun lover. Now I know one of the reasons why I love the sun so much. Sunlight stimulates release of serotonin in the paper. Sunshine serotonin and skin. A partial explanation for seasonal patterns in psychopathology.

They state that human skin has an inherent serotonergic system. Their peers capable of generating serotonin and the machinery of the serotonergic system is present in the skin. For example, tryptophan hydroxy lays, the initial enzyme in the Synthesis. Serotonin is found in the human skin and scared of getting skin cancer because we hear so much about it in the news. But the disease burden from too little sun is far higher than the disease burden from too much sun.

When we get too little sun bones do not form properly, we get depressed, and we frequently get sick. This is probably because we get to the level of the extremely important vitamin D a Swedish study found that sufficient levels of vitamin D in early life were correlated with a decreased risk of developing Type 1 diabetes and a Finnish study found that children who got 2000 IU of Vitamin D per day, the equivalent of 50 micrograms, from the age of 1 and 80 percent lower risk for developing Type 1 diabetes later in life.

There are even some indications that Vitamin D can help prevent multiple sclerosis. There are certain factors that influence vitamin D production. Some of the most important ones are the time spent in the sun. How high the sun is in the sky.

Clothes women wear a burka are often vitamin D deficient excess fat in the body sunscreen and skin melanin summed up the efficiency of production depends on the number of UVB photons and penetrate the skin. The author states that for most white people a half hour in the sun and a bathing suit can initiate the release. Fifty thousand international units are one point twenty-five milligrams of Vitamin D into the circulation within 24 hours of exposure.

The same amount of exposure to 20000 30000 international units in 10 individuals and 8000 to 10000 internationals units and dark-skinned people if the mood is down and the sun is up. Get outside and let the sunlight and enjoy the extra serotonin as we know from the first section. Vitamin D also increases your level of dopamine giving you an extra nudge in your mood.

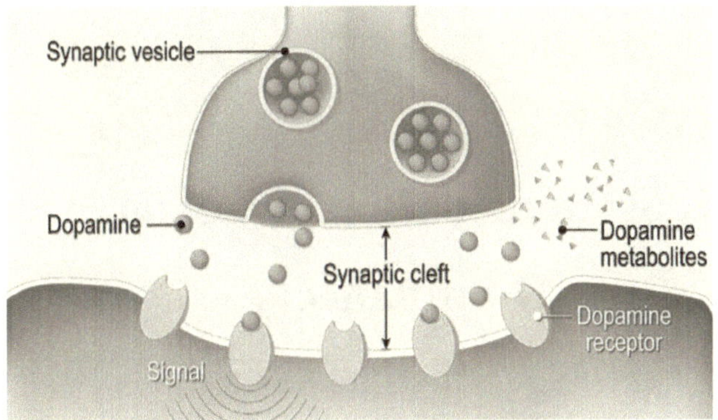

Boost Serotonin with Social Dominance

Why does it feel so good when others admire you. And give you respect. Why do you get that calm certain feeling that everything will be OK. A significant part of that answer lies in semi-tone the study neural mechanisms of social dominance.

Look at how the social status of monkeys affected their serotonin level and vice versa. They stated that dominant monkeys are approximately twice the serotonin concentrations of ordinate monkeys. However, the serotonin levels of dominant monkeys were very sensitive to the presence of subordinate's when that dominant monkey was taken out of the social context. It's serotonin level went down to about the same as that of the subordinates.

Then one day this shows us that serotonin really is a social chemical and that its level is highly correlated with hierarchical status further. They stated that the transition from a subordinate to a dominant position in the social hierarchy was accompanied by an increase in serotonin levels. It has been shown that you can change the social hierarchy of monkeys by changing their serotonin levels after removing the dominant monkey from the group.

They get some of the same ordinate monkeys trip the fan to elevate their serotonin or oxytocin to inhibit re-uptake the treated monkeys then went on to become more dominant than the untreated control group. When they instead gave the monkeys, the serotonin lowering drug that treated monkeys get away any dominance to the untreated control group.

The findings indicate that there is two-way interaction between serotonin and social dominance increased serotonin increases dominance and increased dominance increases serotonin levels studies were also done in humans. Like they said in the study administration of serotonin to humans has a similar effect on social dominance.

Healthy human participants received a dose of tryptophan of three grams per day with their meals for 12 days and were asked to verbally describe their own communication frequency agreeableness dominance. The participants who had been administered tryptophan exhibited an increase in dominant behavior and a decrease in quarrelsome behavior meaning critical comments of others social dominance can sound harsh.

Many of us will probably get negative associations by hearing this term. There is nothing inherently negative with social dominance However we instinctively seek the leadership of others in some situations in other situations. We take on leadership ourselves social dominance does not even have to include great physical strength and size.

Like they say in the study in animal societies physical strength tends to determine social rank but in human societies it is not only physical strength but also cognitive factors such as intelligence and emotional stability that determines his or her social ranking. One interesting thing the study found was that we used facial expressions of others to evaluate social rank. This makes sense in more than one way.

We tend to like what makes us feel good and a calm happy face makes us feel calmer and happier and anxious or scared face makes us feel more anxious and scared which we don't like or at least won't follow. In the study effects of self-generated facial expressions and mood they found the participant's experience increased positive moods when they engaged in positive facial expressions and decreased positive moods when they engaged in negative facial expressions.

Effect was stronger when they also looked at themselves in the mirror and the effect was the strongest and self-conscious individuals' defects were equally strong in men and women. This means that you can increase your social dominance by self-generating the facial expressions of a typically socially dominant person. Your mood will follow which again makes it easier to generate the facial expressions.

This is an effect that has been repeatedly shown in Cognitive Neuroscience and is called priming another way to use priming is to internally say the words that you associate with the good feelings. You want to feel one way to tie all this together is to use both facial and word priming at the same time. Let's say three typical feelings are behaviors of socially dominant people is to be bold excited and focused.

You can say those three words inside while trying to change your face to that of a person who embodies these three qualities rotate the words in your mind while adjusting your facial expressions. For extra effect you can do this while looking into a mirror. You will feel more socially dominant which in turn increases your serotonin which in turn increases your social dominance. When something throws you off balance you can go right back to this technique. You can use this technique to generate any feeling you desire. The effect is usually not enormous, but you will definitely feel a change.

There are more studies that have looked at how trip the fans effect on serotonin levels can increase social dominance and agreeable behavior in the study. The role of serotonin and human mood and social interaction. Insights from Alter to the walls. They state that preliminary data indicate a trip.

The fan also increases dominant behavior during social interactions over all studies manipulating trip the family will support the idea that low serotonin can predispose subjects to mood and impulse control disorders. Higher levels of serotonin may help to promote more constructive social interactions by decreasing aggression and increasing dominance and in the study tryptophan serotonin and human social behavior.

They say that animal research suggests that increasing serotonin can decrease aggression increase affiliated behaviors and increase dominant behaviors. We tested the relevance of these data to humans by giving hundred healthy people tryptophan. One gram after each meal and placebo each for 12 days in a double-blind crossover study. Social behaviors were studied using an advanced sampling method in which subjects filled in a one-page questionnaire about their behaviors.

After each social interaction lasting at least five minutes and cost a significant decrease in quarrelsome behavior and a significant increase in dominant behaviors. So, we see that not only do we get more serotonin when you are socially dominant. Serotonin also makes you more socially dominant and we also see that being more socially dominant in general makes you more agreeable less aggressive and more inclined to cooperate and associate with others.

Boost Serotonin with Meditation

Serotonin is thought to be one of the main reasons why we feel so calm and peaceful after a session of meditation serotonin has been called the breast and fulfillment hormone as opposed to being in the highly stressful fight or flight mode.

Anecdotal evidence says for a long-time supported meditation as a treatment for anxiety this randomized control trial looked at how mindfulness compares to normal treatments for generalized anxiety disorder a disorder of chronic worry and hyper arousal 93 individuals were randomized to an eight-week intervention of either a mindfulness-based stress reduction program or through stress management education program the mindfulness-based program worked significantly better than the stress management program in reducing safety.

And four of the skills on the last and the scales both lent significant reductions in anxiety but there was no significant difference between the two authors of the study speculated that this was because this particular scale heavily was bodily symptoms and is insensitive to psychological changes.

The mindfulness-based program also led to the greatest increase in positive self-statements this study looked at how cell meditation affected the interior prefrontal cortex and the certain nervous system. They used EEG to correlate the changes in brain activity with changes in serotonin levels.

The author states EEG revealed increased Alpha band activity and decreased theta band activity during tendon breathing age changes recorded or with a significant increase in whole blood serotonin levels. These results suggest that activation of the interior prefrontal cortex and serotonin system may be responsible for the improvement of negative mood. An EEG signal changes served during tandem breathing some researchers have also found a correlation between meditation serotonin and visual hallucinations.

When serotonin inhibits the lateral nucleus a relay center in the visual pathway of the thalamus it reduces the transmission of visual information. The absence of sensory stimulus leads to internally generated imagery this resolved in visual hallucinations similar to the effects of certain nerve drugs like LSD and psilocybin as we saw in the previous section.

Meditation also improves our levels of dopamine serotonin can interact with dopamine and enhance feelings of euphoria. Often experience from meditation is associated with large increases in the sleep promoting hormone melatonin which can be synthesize from serotonin in the pineal gland activation of the pineal gland.

Meditation can also lead to the release of the powerful hallucinogen, DMT, a structural analogue to serotonin and melatonin like the authors of this study States meditation is associated with a sharp increase of classman melatonin stimulation of the pineal gland by the lateral hypothalamus is responsible for the heightened melatonin decreased melatonin may result in the calmness and decreased awareness of pain seen during meditation.

It is also noted that during heightened activation pineal enzymes synthesize five Methos see dimethyl tryptamine VMT which is a powerful hallucinogen several studies have linked TMT to out-of-body experience. Time-Space distortion and other such mystical states.

Boost Serotonin with Exercise

The connection between exercise and a good mood is clear exercise has been shown to have both antidepressant and anxiolytic effects a possible reason for this is that exercise increases the firing rates of serotonin neurons. This results in an increase of serotonin release and synthesis.

Another reason why exercise boosts your serotonin is that there is an increase of the serotonin building block tryptophan in your brain that persists after exercise. This is because exercise leads to a decrease in your blood levels of brand chained amino acids. This is important because branching amino acids compete with the fat to cross the blood brain barrier.

Also, when we exercise, we start breaking down fat molecules these fat molecules compete with tryptophan for slots and transborder proteins. This leads to an increase of tripped the fan in the blood. So, exercise elevated blood tryptophan and decreases its competition in crossing the blood brain barrier. Once a fan has reached the brain it is immediately put to use in building certain exercise also boosts your levels of another brain chemical called brain derived neuro tropic factor.

BNF which stimulates release of serotonin will come back to being asked later in the book. Our ancestors didn't run or want to look fit and Bragg at the office about their personal records. They moved to hunt and gather food. This is also in their brains needed to function optimally. This is probably some of the reason why exercise has evolved to become such a potent stimulator of neurotransmitters.

Our genes are encoded for exercise in a bookstore. Dr. John J. Ratty advises this exercise like our ancestors walk and jog clocks run a couple of times a week and go for the kill. Every now and then by sprinting all out. But if we exercise for 30 minutes every day of the week, we would still be moving less than half the amount. Our genes are encoded for.

However, the most important thing is to start. If you can't stand the thought of exercising start with five minutes of walking outside per day, then slowly work yourself up to what exercise physiologist. Brian does chef from Duke University says it's the optimal level of exercise some form of aerobic exercise six days a week for 45 to 60 minutes. It might take you a couple of years to reach this level over that time slowly and gradually increasing exercise. You will continuously improve your brain chemistry.

Boost Serotonin with Thought

Some researchers have found that thoughts affect our serotonin levels they use positron emission tomography to measure serotonin levels in people went through positive negative and neutral mood inductions when they reported higher mood levels their serotonin production was higher in the anterior cingulate cortex when they reported lower levels serotonin production was lower.

This means that the interaction between serotonin and mood is two-way serotonin influences mood and mood influences serotonin. Anything that spikes your mood spikes your serotonin to get this effect you can use the priming trick from the chapter on serotonin and social dominance. Say three words they use sociate with good feelings and put on the facial expression you associate with those good feelings.

Boost Serotonin with Vitamins

There has not been done much clinical research and Vitamin B3 or niacin effect on anxiety. However, there is some anecdotal evidence for its potency. Jonathan E. Prose is a professor at the Canadian College of Natural pathic medicine. He presented three case studies in the paper supplemental niacinamide mitigates inside symptoms three case reports three of his patients lost much or all of their anxiety in high doses of niacinamide niacin can have an effect on the side in several ways.

You might have a nice deficiency. You can have benzodiazepine like effects because of its effect on the neurotransmitter GABA and it could be because it raises serotonin levels by diverting tryptophan to serotonin production vitamin D 6 or paradox has been found to increase serotonin levels in monkeys' paradox and is a B vitamin that is cheap and widely available you can get both niacin and paradox in from vitamin B complex together with many other important B-vitamins.

Boost Serotonin with Theanine

See an in an amino acid fountain you can enter our brain and affect our levels of neurotransmitters. CNN seems to elevate our brain levels of both dopamine and serotonin. Like they say in this study see an administration cause significant increases in serotonin and or dopamine concentrations in the brain especially in the striatum hypothalamus and hippocampus.

Direct administration of Theanine and into brain striatum by micro injection caused a significant increase of dopamine release in a dose deepen manner. And in this study, they say that Health eon has been historically reported as a relaxing agent prompting scientific research on his pharmacology animal new chemistry studies suggests that healthy increases brain serotonin dopamine and GABA levels.

In addition, it has been shown to exert neuroprotective effects and behavioral studies in animals just improvement in learning and memory. However, there is some controversy on thinning's effect on serotonin. One study found that injecting CNN into rat's brains lowered serotonin levels try drinking green tea or taking a scene in supplement to see if CNN has a good effect on you.

Boost Serotonin with Omega 3

The most important maigre 3 fatty acids are EPA and DHEA EPA has been proposed to increase serotonin release and DNJ influences serotonin receptors by increasing cell membrane fluidity long term Omega 3 intakes can increase your serotonin levels like this statin this study. It has been reported that higher concentrations of plasma DHEA predict an increase in serotonergic neurotransmission in healthy adults and in an experimental animal model of depression.

Conversely Omega 3 deficiency results in an increase of serotonin receptor density in the frontal cortex probably due to an adaptation to reduce serotonergic function. If you're a vegan, you can still get maigre three from Plan through like flaxseeds and Chia plant-based omega 3 is in the form of alcohol in the Lining acid. But it can be converted to EPA and DHEA. However, the conversion is slow.

Further the conversion from ala to DHEA and EPA is reduced when the intake of Omega 6 is high. A good alternative for billions algae-based Omega 3 oil.

Boost Serotonin with Gut Bacteria

Gut gets filled with bacteria both good and bad gut flora out of balance can have a wide range of negative effects on your health your brain health and mood is also affected. One study found the probiotic by fear of bacteria infanticide significantly increased levels of tryptophan in the blood.

They say that the attenuation of pro inflammatory immune responses and the elevation of the serotonergic precursor trick to found by Fitow bacteria treatment provides encouraging evidence in support of the proposition that this probiotic may possess antidepressant properties.

Probiotic treatment over eight we said and found to help lower depression some of the reasons for this might be increased serotonin production or good bacteria can increase by taking a probiotic supplement or eating probiotic food like sauerkraut and kimchi or good bacteria need prebiotic fiber. Some good sources of probiotics are onions leek garlic Jerusalem artichoke and asparagus.

Boost Serotonin by Improving Thyroid Function

Your thyroid regulates an enormous number of processes in your body. If your thyroid is dysfunctional you can fall into depression. It's also associated with a whole range of other mental problems. And thyroid hormone serotonin and mood of synergy and significance in the brain. They say that Disorders of the thyroid gland are frequently associated with severe mental disturbances.

It is well established that thyroid hormones are essential for both the development and maturation of the human brain affecting such diverse events as neuronal processing and integration. Glial cell proliferation Miley nation and the synthesis of QI and science required for neurotransmitter synthesis some other symptoms of a dysfunctional thyroid include metabolic syndrome and cold intolerance weight gain.

And this study they say that small differences in thyroid function are associated with up to five kilograms difference in body weight the amount of energy we use for resting is high in hyperthyroidism and low in hypo thyroid Asom inflammatory bowel disease. Note that for some of these symptoms it's difficult to know which is cause and which is effect.

It could also be that both are effects of a deeper problem. Carotid arterial plucking and strokes hair loss dry skin infertility and reproductive dysfunction and weakened immune system the thyroid also affects our production of serotonin plasma serotonin levels have been shown to correlate positively with T-3 thyroid hormone concentration. Also, the synthesis of serotonin tends to be high in cases of hyperthyroidism and low in cases of hypothyroidism.

And this study they state that the influence of the thyroid system on neurotransmitters particularly serotonin and norepinephrine which putatively play a major role in the regulation of mood and behavior may contribute to the mechanisms of mood modulation and in this study, they say that thyroid hormone at location of euthyroid proteins increased cortical or wholegrain serotonin 5 HTP and 5 8 IJA concentrations in 10 studies begin by healing your gut when you have a leaky gut.

Large proteins into your bloodstream some of these proteins like gliadin which is a component of gluten or very similar to the tissue in your thyroid when your immune system attacks these invading proteins. It also attacks your thyroid irritable bowel syndrome tends to be associated with leads you get to heal you get is important to stay away from foods you are allergic or sensitive to in this study they say that there is a recognized association between the symptoms of IBS food hypersensitivity and in some cases true food allergy when intestinal permeability was measured pre and post provocation with suspect foods.

It was demonstrated that these patients developed abnormal permeability try to avoid pro-inflammatory foods as much as you possibly can. These include modern foods like refined flours sugar and high fructose corn syrup and industrial oils high in omega 6. You might notice what all these foods have in common. They have all been invented recently.

Our bodies haven't adapted yet. There also seems to be a link between insulin resistance and diabetes and thyroid dysfunction. In this study they say that the frequency of thyroid dysfunction diabetic patients is higher than that of the general population and up to a third of patients with type 1 diabetes ultimately develop thyroid dysfunction insulin resistance and most cases of diabetes are caused by excessive amounts of refined flours sugar and high fructose corn syrup.

My best tips for increasing your thyroid function neurotransmitter levels and overall health are limit sugar and other refined carbohydrates. The absolute minimum state to delicious whole foods. The next step is to get adequate amounts of important vitamins and minerals. Start by optimizing your IRA levels together with selenium iodine and selenium works together in the thyroid in this study dietary iodine and selenium interact to affect thyroid hormone metabolism of rats.

They say that high iodine intake when selenium is deficient may permit thyroid tissue damage. And in this study, they say that adequate selenium nutrition supports efficient thyroid hormone synthesis and metabolism and protects the thyroid gland from damage by excessive iodide exposure. In regents of combined severe iodine and selenium deficiency normalization of iodine supply is mandatory for initiation of selenium supplementation in order to prevent hypothyroidism. Selenium supplementation has also been shown to help in our immune thyroid diseases like Hashimoto's disease Graves' disease.

Vitamin D is another important vitamin which we have discussed several times in this book. There is a significantly higher prevalence of vitamin D deficiency in people with autoimmune thyroid disease. This study they say that low levels of vitamin D have also been associated with thyroid disease such as Hashimoto's Thyroiditis.

Similarly, patients with new onset Graves' disease were found to have decreased 25 hydroxy Vitamin D concentrations another vitamin which might be important is vitamin B-12. The next step is reducing the stress in your life. Stress is associated with autoimmune viral diseases practice stress management and relaxation techniques.

If you haven't tried meditation, I recommend that we have multiple signs that techniques for regaining your inner peace in our corps mastery in a piece a quick fix for stress levels that will work wonders for 90 percent of the population is the batch email and cell phone use. Close your email. Put away your phone. Most of the day only check them once or three times a day.

If you want some stress management until form the amino acid tyrosine might be what you're looking for. These researchers funded stressed out mice had significantly decreased levels of thyroid hormones tyrosine supplementation significantly increased levels of thyroid hormones.

They say that after four weeks of chronic stress dopamine and nor epinephrine levels and the pallium hippocampus and hypothalamus were significantly decreased levels of dopamine in the pallium and hippocampus as well as levels of norepinephrine and the pallium and the thalamus restored by L. tyrosine supplementation.

Lastly, we have alcohol in this study impact of alcohol use on thyroid function. They say that alcohol has been reported to cause direct suppression of thyroid function by cellular toxicity and indirect suppression by blunting firetrap in releasing hormone response. It causes a decrease of peripheral thyroid hormones during chronic use and in withdrawal.

And that's the effect of alcohol on the hypothermic pituitary thyroid axis is significant. And alcohol consumption affects almost all aspects of the functioning of the thyroid gland. Given the co-morbidity of mood disorders in alcoholism and the relation of mood disorders with hypothyroidism these findings open up interesting theoretical possibilities to explain the increased occurrence of mood disorders and alcoholism.

To conclude, stay away from foods you are allergic or sensitive to. Limit modern foods to the absolute minimum. This is everything that includes refined flour sugar and high fructose corn syrup and industrial oils sign Omega says basically the middle aisles in supermarkets and grocery stores. A lot of these food items can sit on the shelf for months or years without rotting set in another way.

Stick to the delicious whole foods. Some of you will also benefit from ditching all kinds of corn products like bread and cereal. Get adequate levels of both iodine and selenium. Some sources of iodine are iodine rich salt and seafood in general but especially kelp Brazil nuts are packed with selenium and 4:58 nuts are more than enough per day.

You can also get your item and selenium from supplements get enough vitamin D from sun exposure and supplementation. Most people need supplementation in winter some needed even in summer. The same goes with vitamin B-12. A lot of people are deficient, and supplements are teeth Wiig and especially need to supplement with B-12 become master of your own stress levels.

Tyrosine supplements might help ease some of the way. And lastly limit your alcohol consumption if you want to learn more about the thyroid. I recommend reading Chris aggressor's blog posts on thyroid dysfunction. But do a fact check before you do anything drastic. You should do the same for this book. Thank you for watching.

The Feeling of Endorphins

Endorphins are the feeling of euphoria after a great workout. They make you feel relaxed fulfilled safe warm and happy. The name endorphins come from the term and Detin is morphine and dodginess means that they are produced by our body endorphins or opiates like medical morphine and heroin. The most well-known endorphin produced by the body is highly potent.

This study states on a smaller basis better endorphin is 18 to thirty-three times more potent than morphine. It is however produced in fairly small quantities unlike medical morphine and heroin. Endorphins are not highly addictive and the consequences of having say a minor exercise addiction are mostly positive by inhibiting the sending of pain signals endorphins main task is to mask pain.

They function through various mechanisms in both the central and peripheral nervous system to relieve pain. When bound to their new opioid receptors they helped early humans escape from lions and other dangers. In prehistoric times because they let you run fast and long without getting overwhelmed by pain, they gave us a good feeling.

After spending long hours chasing prey or gathering food and motivated us to repeat that behavior endorphins help you learn more effectively and to remember what you have learned in our day and age. We can take advantage of this when we want to learn new skills or create new habits. One study state that endorphins cause amnesia for extraneous details of a task allowing focusing on Main Events and prevent the extinction of a learned task.

Another study says that endogenous opioids seem to have important effects upon memory endorphins make your brain more susceptible to change and making new conditioned responses. The study endorphins in learning states that a number of learning paradigms for example the conditioned emotional response preference for signal shock condition taste aversions and learned helplessness were presented in support of this mediation of learning by the endorphins.

This means that you can stimulate the release of endorphins when you want to create new habits endorphins can also postpone cerebral aging of the brain and boost your immune system ensuring that you stay healthy and feel good. This group of chemicals is involved in the good feelings you get from a good tasting meal.

Laughing meditating making and listening to music drinking moderate amounts of alcohol having sex getting massages and getting sunlight. Among other things going for too long without endorphins will result in an imbalance and a whole range of negative effects on both mental and physical health. The most effective ways to stimulate release of endorphins will be covered in this section of the book.

The Feeling of Low Endorphin Levels

Low endorphin levels are associated with several negative effects on mental and physical health. A meta-analysis of several studies on migraine found a decrease in better endorphin levels in sufferers of both chronic and episodic migraine.

People with chronic pain conditions in general including fibromyalgia have lower than normal levels of endorphins low endorphin levels are associated with obesity. Aging of the brain diabetes and psychiatric diseases like depersonalization disorder based on these studies we can assume that having low endorphin levels does not promote good feelings.

Boost Endorphins with Exercise

You have probably heard of the term runner's high this euphoric high that you get after a hard workout is mostly due to endorphin release. It is often accompanied by a positive and energized outlook on life. Regular exercise is the most well-known way to stimulate the release of endorphins.

Seemingly the higher the intensity of the exercise the more endorphins you get. The study endorphins and exercise say that elevated Seram better endorphin concentrations induced by exercise have been linked to several psychological and physiological changes including mood state changes and exercise induced euphoria.

Endorphins make exercise more easily doable by relieving pain and rewarding you with a good feeling that makes you want to repeat the behavior. It is a well-known fact that exercise is good for you it strengthens your heart lowers blood pressure increases energy levels strengthens your bones and makes you look healthier.

Regular exercise has also been proven to reduce stress reduce feelings of anxiety and depression boosts self-esteem and improve sleep endorphins are part of the explanation for most of these benefits. Exercise keeps your body in mind young and feeling good. We also know that exercise promotes growth of new brain cells especially in the hippocampus the area responsible for emotions memory and the autonomous nervous system.

The study exercised induced for motion of hippocampal cell proliferation requires better endorphin states that endorphins are required for the growth of new brain cells in response to exercise it concludes that the endorphin release during running is a key factor for exercise induced cell proliferation. The benefits of regular exercise are obvious whoever you are you should aim to do some kind of regular exercise.

Find something that you enjoy. It does not have to be super intense. You can go for a walk do yoga play golf swim lift weights run climb your imagination sets the limits you could even combine the exercise with what you learn in the dopamine section. Set exercise goals and make plans for how you will get a good boost of endorphins by doing some kind of exercise that you enjoy.

Planning a task and finishing it will give you a dopamine boost. The exercise itself will give you endorphins exercise can also include socialization which means there are several opportunities to boost both Serotonin and oxytocin as well giving you a complete cocktail of happiness boosting neurochemicals.

Boost Endorphins with Laughter

You have probably experienced laughing so hard that you would almost prefer to stop because of the stomach pain bluffing is technically internal convulsions which would be painful if not for endorphins. In fact, the endorphins released when you laugh will increase your pain threshold for a while. Laughter makes you feel better and happier which in turn affects your health.

The expression a good laugh prolongs life even seems to be scientifically valid. A link between laughter and improved cardiovascular health was found in the study. The effect of mirthful laughter on the human cardiovascular system even expecting to laugh can boost your endorphins. This study States in its title that better endorphin and HGH increase are associated with both the anticipation and experience of mirthful laughter.

It goes on to say we have also reported that anticipation of a behavioral after eustress or beneficial stress event increases positive psychological mood states. Prior to the intervention and that these findings have immune modulation implications that may be beneficial in stress reduction for wellness and prevention.

In other words, laughter or the anticipation of it promotes good health and reduces stress. Some studies on humans are based on self-reporting of positive emotional states. The findings in the study. Laughing rats are optimistic. Confirm that laughter induced measurable positive emotion in rats akin to human joy to do this.

The researchers tickled a bunch of rats and measured their emotional response. Their findings indicate that tickling induced positive emotions which are directly indexed in rats by laughter can make animals more optimistic. You can set the intention to laugh more often to experience the positive effects of endorphins ranging from anti-depressant effects to physical well-being.

Find out what makes you laugh and do more of it. You can go to comedy clubs watch funny videos have fun with friends or family or laugh with your coworkers. Saying positive words in your head light amused happy laughing etc. can put you in a better mood and prime you to laugh more easily. You can even induce laughter yourself simply by faking it.

Eventually you will not be able not to laugh for real. This is called Laughter Yoga and is practiced around the world. This study on laughter yoga concludes that a large number of Americans regardless of age and physical ability could benefit from laughter yoga laugh more to create the positive spiral of good emotions.

Boost Endorphins with Music

Music affects endorphin levels according to this study. Musical activities like singing and dancing are associated with higher levels of endorphins. This meteor analysis suggests that active engagement in musical activities for example vigorous singing dancing or drumming results in greater endorphin activation than passive listening.

One study found that listening to techno music is accompanied by a significant increase in better endorphin. The reason is thought to be because of its strong rhythmic beads and engagement of motor regions of the brain. The same study detected no significant changes from listening to classical music.

Another study found that relaxation following music listening is associated with endorphins. The meta-analysis states that as indicated by the evidence reviewed above the way that we experience music whether during passive listening or active engagement appears to involve and dodginess opioid system and endorphins specifically listen to music you enjoy dance sing and drum if you feel like it. Create music. If you're into that the more active your role in musical activities the more endorphins, you seem to get.

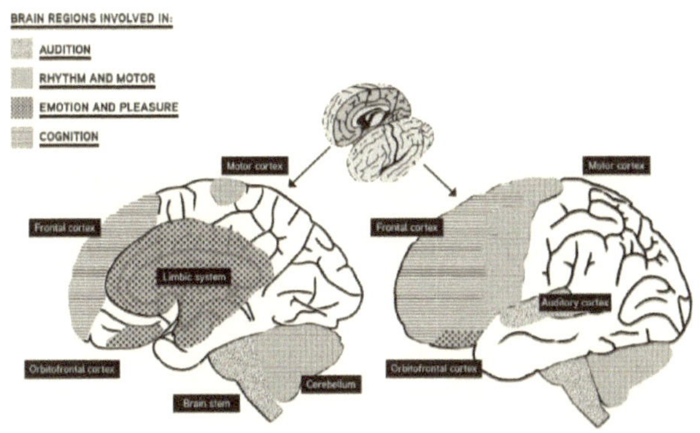

Boost Endorphins with Sunlight

The some may be best known for boosting production of vitamin D. And as we saw in the previous chapters. Serotonin but the sun's ultraviolet rays also increase blood levels of endorphins. The study benefits of sunlight a bright spot for human health says that melanocytes in human skin express a fully functioning endorphin receptor system and that the cutaneous pigment system is important stress response element of the skin.

In other words, sunlight boosts endorphins because it stresses the skin just like exercise boosts endorphins due to physiological stress. Sunlight has several physiologic effects on the skin including altering the immune system and increasing production of nitric oxide and chemical that we will discuss later on. Get out in the sun for up to an hour every day. Just make sure you don't get burned if you stay any longer.

The Feeling of GABA

Think back to a time when you were handling complex and stressful situations like a champ you were solved an intense event and immediately put it behind you without dwelling on it or overthinking it a reason for this type of behavior is GABA or Dema amino butyric acid. GABA it's a calming inhibitory neurotransmitter. It puts the brakes on brain activity when needed.

It's like valium produced by your body GABA doesn't get as much attention as the other inhibitory neurotransmitter serotonin but it's just as important for your mental well-being. It enables your brain to put an end to persistent negative thoughts circulating in your mind. Adequate GABA and serotonin activity in the brain leads to a stable calm feeling. With sufficient GABA levels calm social behavior eye contact quality sleep and healthy bowel function.

Being deficient in GABA might lead to increased worry and stress. Racing thoughts might keep you up at night and your heart might beat a radically. The best ways to boost GABA naturally will be covered in this section of the book.

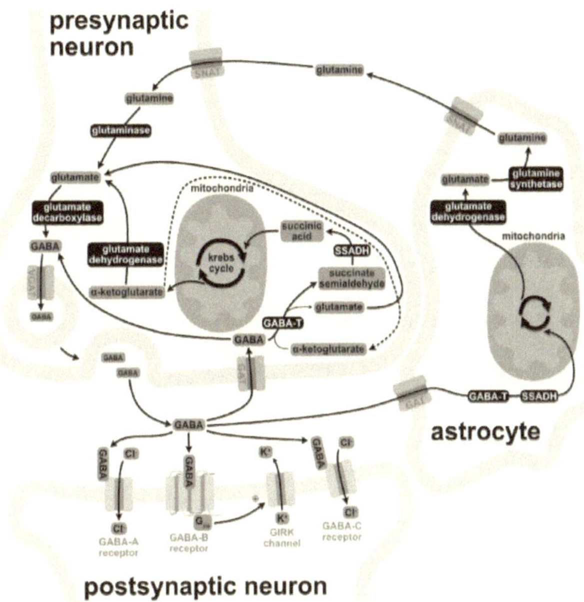

presynaptic neuron
glutamine
SNAT
glutamine
glutaminase
glutamate
glutamate decarboxylase
GABA
GAT
GABA
GABA
glutamate dehydrogenase
α-ketoglutarate
mitochondria
krebs cycle
succinic acid
SSADH
succinate semialdehyde
glutamate
GABA-T
GABA
α-ketoglutarate
GAT
GABA
GABA
GABA
Cl
Cl
GABA
K
GABA
Cl
Cl
G
K
Cl
GABA-A receptor
GABA-B receptor
GIRK channel
GABA-C receptor
postsynaptic neuron
glutamine
SNAT
glutamine
glutamate
glutamine synthetase
glutamate dehydrogenase
mitochondria
GAT
GABA-T
SSADH
astrocyte

The Feeling of Low GABA Levels

Imagine feeling depressed anxious stressed-out having trouble sleeping and having a poor immune system these are some of the common symptoms associated with low levels. Not only are there several studies linking low carb levels to all of the above symptoms but a deficiency in GABA may also lead to many other problems.

Because GABA is the main inhibitor in neurotransmitter it helps keep calm and it puts the brakes on brain activity when needed. Research indicates that a deficiency in GABA may lead to hypertension, atherosclerosis, motion sickness, digestive disorders, ADHD, epileptic seizures, panic disorders, Tourette's syndrome, bronchitis and low growth hormone levels.

If you are experiencing any of these symptoms it could be worthwhile to investigate whether you have a deficiency in double levels. You can take our online neurotransmitter test to get an indication a link is included in this lessens resource. Deficiency or not the tips included in the lessons of this section may help you increase your GABA levels and thus your well-being.

Boost GABA with Exercise

Exercise has been mentioned frequently in this book and for good reason. The neurochemical cocktail released during exercise is highly potent making exercise one of the most reliable long term mood boosters ever. When it comes to exercise and GABA, the most interesting study to date is an imaging study from 2016. It comes from a research team at UC Davis health system and shows that exercise increases levels of both GABA and glutamate.

Two of the most abundant neurotransmitters in the brain intense exercise is the most energy demanding activity of the brain encounters more so than calculus or chess. Apparently one of the things the brain is doing with all that energy is making more neurotransmitters. The researchers studied 38 healthy adults who exercised on a stationary bicycle reaching around 85 percent of their maximum heart rate.

The researchers measured glutamate and GABA through several imaging studies using a state-of-the-art powerful MRI scanner. The measurements were done in two different parts of the brain immediately before and after three vigorous exercise sessions lasting between eight and twenty minutes. The same measurements were made on a controlled group who did not exercise levels of glutamate and GABA increased in the exercisers but not in the control group.

The UC Davis NEWSROOM reported that significant increases were found in the visual cortex which processes visual information and the anterior cingulate cortex which helps regulate heart rates some cognitive functions and a motion these findings indicate that exercise could be used as an alternative in treating depression and anxiety. In follow up studies the research team wants to test whether less intense activities such as walking can have similar effects.

If you want to replicate the exercise intensity and duration from the study, you should aim for reaching around 85 percent of your maximum heart rate for eight to 20 minutes. Not that you should be in good shape and good health. Before doing this if you have a heart rate monitor of some sort. You can monitor your heart rate during exercise.

As a general rule you can assume that your maximum heart rate is two hundred and twenty minus your age. For example, if you're 30 years old. Subtract 30 from 220 to get a maximum heart rate of ninety five percent of this would be around and 60. If you don't have a heart rate monitor, you can use burden's talk test when you exercise at an intensity where you are only able to express two- or three-word thoughts.

You generally should be around 80 to 85 percent of your maximum heart rate. It might not be absolutely necessary with such high intensity exercise for similar brain benefits. There are already some interesting studies showing that GABA is increased through less vigorous exercise pacifically yoga. More on this in the next video.

Boost GABA with Yoga

The ancient practice of yoga has been proven effective for reducing symptoms in a variety of disorders including inside the depression and epilepsy these disorders are all associated with low levels of GABA and the symptoms can be reduced by substances known to increase GABA system activity. The 2007 pilot study showed that brain levels of GABA was increased by 27 percent after a 60

Minute session of yoga this study was done on experienced yoga practitioners.

The researchers wanted to find out if the changes in doubles were specific to yoga or whether they could arise from a walking session with similar intensity. In 2010 they published the study effects of yoga versus walking and mood in society and brain Gebel levels. A randomized controlled MRSA study they showed death Iyengar yoga this time practice by beginners increased brain GABA levels whereas walking did not.

The yoga group also reported greater improvement mood and greater decrease in anxiety than walking group. This indicates that higher brain gabbles improve mood and decreases anxiety. The yoga group had only been doing yoga for 12 weeks and saw an increase in brain Galba levels by 13 percent. They experienced yoga practitioners in the first study saw a 27 percent increase around twice as much as the beginners.

Thus, the effects seemed to increase with experience. For those of you want to go deeper. Here are some more studies and a look at some of the mechanisms that might be responsible for yoga's effects and double levels the parasympathetic nervous system is said simply a part of your nervous system that calms and relaxes you.

Yoga's effect GABA levels may be connected with yoga's ability to increase activity in the parasympathetic nervous system the way yoga does. This seems to be in part through stimulating and nerve called the vagas nerve and it is suggested that vagus Nerve Stimulation stimulates release of GABA.

Boost GABA with a Ketogenic Diet

The Ketogenic diet is a diet very low in carbohydrates low to moderate in protein and high in fat. There are many studies showings that a kilo genic diet can help you lose weight and improve health many studies indicate that lifestyle diseases such as diabetes cancer epilepsy heart disease and all Simmers disease can be avoided by a ketogenic diet.

Ketogenic diet means that your intake of carbs is low enough and your intake of fat high enough to put your body in a state called ketosis. This is when fat is turned into ketones in the liver ketone supply energy for the body and brain. In this state your body becomes incredibly efficient at burning fat for energy including excess body fat most bodies are used to burning sugar for energy, most modern bodies.

That is our meat-eating low carb dieting hunter gatherer ancestors spent most of their time in ketosis Aikido genic diet seems to have beneficial effects on the brain one of which is that it can boost levels of GABA. GABA is made from another neurotransmitter, glutamate. These two neurotransmitters are opposites.

Since GABA is the major inhibitory neurotransmitter, and glutamate is the major excitatory neurotransmitter, GABA calms your glutamate that excites you. We need them both.

But too much glutamate is neurotoxic and can cause trouble and in extreme cases it can lead to seizures. This is connected to the body of research showing how epileptic seizures can be avoided by ketogenic diet glutamate can become both GABA, which is inhibitory, and aspartate which is excitatory and neurotoxic.

In excess ketogenic diet seems to favor glutamate becoming GABA instead of aspartate. Science is not yet able to give a complete answer as to why this is, but part of the answer lies in how ketones are metabolized. Agito acetate. One of the ketones becomes glutamine an essential precursor to GABA studies in rats have shown that ketone bodies can increase the carbon content in the rat brain.

And in this study on humans a ketogenic diet was associated with elevated levels of GABA and some but not all subjects studied. A general guideline for the Ketogenic diet is that at least 75 percent of your calories are coming from fat around 20 percent from protein and only around 5 percent from carbohydrates. This is very controverting to a mainstream diet that is extremely high in carbs.

A lot of it from refined sugars getting into ketosis takes at least a few days and it may take a few weeks before you start getting used to it and up to a year for the body to become fully adapted to using fat as fuel this initial induction phase into ketosis is usually accompanied by some discomfort. This is called Keto flu.

And the symptoms can range from nothing at all to mild discomfort and dizziness to full on flu like symptoms for example headaches nausea fatigue cramps and diarrhea. More on this and how to avoid it below. There are a lot of interesting research on the ketogenic diet and its health benefits. If you're interested in learning more about how telegenic diet works and its benefits.

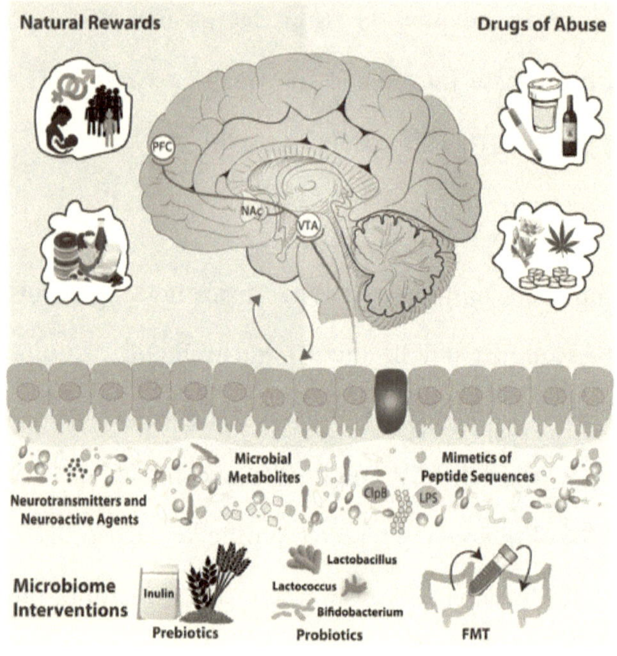

Natural Rewards
Drugs of Abuse
PFC
NAc
VTA
Microbial Metabolites
Mimetics of Peptide Sequences
ClpB
LPS
Neurotransmitters and Neuroactive Agents
Microbiome Interventions
Inulin
Prebiotics
Lactobacillus
Lactococcus
Bifidobacterium
Probiotics
FMT

Boost GABA with Zinc

Zinc is an essential trace element that the body uses to maintain health and perform important functions. It helps with hormone production growth and repair Amanté improves immunity facilitates digestion helps prevent acne improves cognitive function and brain health improves mood improves athletic performance and cardiovascular health.

And it is anti-inflammatory. In one review on the importance of Zinc, researchers write that zinc is such a critical element in human health that even a small deficiency is a disaster. It has been found that to low levels of zinc might promoting safety by lowering GABA levels and that zinc supplementation raising GABA levels may help improve anxiety symptoms. In fact, there are numerous studies on its effect on raising devils' levels. So do you get enough slinked the best way to find out is by taking a red blood cell zinc test.

There are some symptoms you can watch out for but these can all be due to something else. Common symptoms include cravings for salty and sweet food anxiety and psychic disorders diarrhea low energy chronic fatigue, infertility, poor immunity, bad memory, inability to focus, slow wound healing, nerve dysfunction, thinning hair and ringing in the ears.

Serious zinc deficiency resulting in growth retardation, hypo-gonadism immune dysfunction and cognitive impairment affects nearly two billion people in the developing world. Sub optimal zinc levels are common in industrialized countries to marginalizing deficiency and suboptimal since status have been recognized in many groups of the population in both less developed and industrialized countries.

The zinc deficiency is widespread in all areas because of nutrient depleted soils and modern high grain diets. Fight AIDS in grains and legumes inhibits zinc absorption and the foods with the highest levels are meat eggs and some seafood especially oysters. This makes vegans and vegetarians especially exposed to zinc deficiency.

Other groups of people that are a higher risk for zinc deficiency include pregnant and lactating women.

Women on birth control pills endurance athletes' alcoholics people with gastrointestinal diseases elderly people and people taking certain medications like diuretics in conclusion. Zinc is an often-forgotten nutritional staple that a lot of people could benefit from getting more off zinc supplements can be a good and inexpensive way to increase your intake.

In general, you should avoid supplements with Zinc Sulphate and zinc oxide and look for supplements with related forms of zinc for better absorption good forms of zinc supplements include things like Holy Night zinc gluconate, zinc acetate and zinc nitrate with studies indicating that zinc by collimate has the best absorption. For more information on how to choose a zinc supplement and dosages see the resources including with this lesson.

Boost GABA with Magnesium

Magnesium is an important mineral that is often missing even in healthy modern diets. Magnesium is necessary in over 600 metabolic functions, yet it is the second most common nutritional deficiency in developed countries. Magnesium depleted soils stress age medications and underlying health conditions all contributed to widespread munition deficiency.

While the magnesium intake has dropped the last 50 years. Rates of anxiety has skyrocketed low levels of munition is associated with a range of disorders including anxiety high blood pressure diabetes and thyroid imbalances. Magnesium enhances the sensitivity and function of the GABA receptors in the brain making it an essential mineral for GABA activity.

This study says that it's possible that magnesium deficiency is the cause of most major depression and related health problems including IQ loss and addiction. Other than by optimizing Jeb activity magnesium alleviates anxiety and stress by reducing stress hormones it is anti-inflammatory and brain inflammation is linked to both anxiety and depression.

It removes heavy metals from the body it increases neuroplasticity to help rewire an anxious brain and it keeps blood sugar levels stable. Nishiyama also boosts the other inhibitory neurotransmitter of serotonin and therefore reduces depression anxiety and depression go hand in hand.

This study states that 85 percent of patients with depression also experience anxiety and that depression occurs in up to 90 percent of patients with anxiety disorders other studies have found that munition was as effective as antidepressants in treating depression and that supplemental magnesium provided recovery from major depression in less than seven days. It seems that almost everyone could benefit from increasing their magnesium intake.

Some of the best food sources of magnesium are Orman's spinach Brazil nuts cashews black beans peanut butter and avocado also magnesium supplements is a good idea to increase your intake of this important mineral. You should look for supplements that include magnesium from several sources the worst sources are magnesium oxide and ignitions sulfate.

The best forms of supplements include magnesium citrate magnesia and vice innate Mallet and magnesium toroid. For more information on how to choose a magnesium supplement and dosages see the resources included with this chapter.

Boost GABA with L-Theanine

Healthy I mean is an amino acid found pretty much exclusively in there. It has been mentioned previously in this book that it increases levels of dopamine and serotonin. It also increases levels of GABA. This study shows that L-Theanine reduces stress and makes you more resilient to whatever life throws your way. Both

GABA and healthy earnings effects is that they change your brain wave activity.

Alpha Waves are associated with deep relaxation and calmness that waves are associated with focus and conscious thought but too much of them may lead to stress and anxiety. Tremor increases alpha waves and decreases better waves. So does the annoying 50 milligrams of healthy is enough to change your brain wave state. The dosages found in a cup of green and black the various from around eight milligrams to 46 milligrams healthy and in supplements do exist.

But the research on their effects is not conclusive. Nevertheless, it proves safe and effective for short term use. One or more cups of high-quality green tea like matter is a good place to start. Green tea is well-studied and have stood the test of time. Studies have found synergistic effects on cognitive function and mood. When the inning and caffeine has been taken together both of these substances are found in green tea alongside a wide range of other beneficial compounds.

Disclaimer

We do not advocate nutritional supplementation over proper medical advice or treatment. This course is not intended to provide diagnosis, treatment or medical advice. Please consult with a physician or other healthcare professional regarding any medical or health related diagnosis or treatment options.

A general guideline for the ketogenic diet is that at least 75% of your calories are coming from fat, around 20% from protein, and only around 5% from carbohydrates. But individual differences on what it takes for each body to start producing ketones will occur. For athletes a slightly higher protein intake may work. And some people can get away with a slightly higher intake of carbs, as well. Intake of medium-chain triglycerides (MCT) might help induce ketosis.

Getting into ketosis takes at least a few days, and it may take a few weeks before you start getting used to it [17], and up to a year for the body to become fully adapted to using fat as fuel.

The initial induction phase into ketosis may last a few days to a couple of weeks, and is usually accompanied by some discomfort. This is called "keto flu" and the symptoms can range from nothing at all, to mild discomfort and dizziness, to full on flu-like symptoms – e.g. headaches, nausea, fatigue, cramps, and diarrhea.

One reason for this is that any major diet alteration is likely to lead to changes in the gut bacterial flora.

Another reason is that when people move from a standard diet to a ketogenic diet they will flush out a lot of retained water, and with it electrolytes. This is due to the high salt content (salt retains water) of processed foods, and the fact that carbohydrates retains a lot of water. Also, lower insulin levels can signal the kidneys to discard excess water. All this tends to increase people's water intake, something that combined with a lower retention will effectively flush electrolytes out.

The possible flu-like symptoms following are only transitory. However, they can be mitigated by increasing intake of sodium, potassium, and magnesium. Without going into great detail, the general consensus among low-carb experts is to aim for something like this:

- 5g of sodium (table salt)

- 1g of potassium

- 300 mg of magnesium

This means you should generously salt your meals with sodium and potassium salts, and take a magnesium supplement. A natural alternative is bone broth, or bouillon.

Other tricks to mitigate possible "keto-flu" is too eat enough fat, add medium-chained triglycerides (MCT) to your diet, and get enough physical activity.

The Ketogenic Diet – Resources:

http://www.ketogenic-diet-resource.com/

https://authoritynutrition.com/ketogenic-diet-101/

http://www.ruled.me/guide-keto-diet/#

http://www.ruled.me/ketogenic-diet-food-list/

http://ketodietapp.com/Blog/post/2015/01/03/Keto-Diet-Food-List-What-to-Eat-and-Avoid

Meat free and vegan:

http://ketomotive.com/vegan-ketogenic-diet/

http://meatfreeketo.com/

http://www.ketosisirl.com/vegan-ketogenic-diet/

Reference list from this lesson:

1. Keogh JB, Brinkworth GD, Noakes M, et al. (2008). Effects of weight loss from a very-low-carbohydrate diet on endothelial function and markers of cardiovascular disease risk in subjects with abdominal obesity. Am J Clin

Nutr 2008;87:567–76.

http://ajcn.nutrition.org/content/87/3/567.long

2. Westman, E. C., Yancy, W. S., Mavropoulos, J. C., Marquart, M., & McDuffie, J. R. (2008). The effect of a low-carbohydrate, ketogenic diet versus a low-glycemic index diet on glycemic control in type 2 diabetes mellitus. Nutrition & Metabolism, 5, 36. http://doi.org/10.1186/1743-7075-5-36

https://www.ncbi.nlm.nih.gov/pmc/articles/PMC2633336/

3. McClernon FJ, Yancy WS Jr, Eberstein JA, Atkins RC, Westman EC. (2007). The effects of a low-carbohydrate ketogenic diet and a low-fat diet on mood, hunger, and other self-reported symptoms. Obesity (Silver

Spring). 2007 Jan;15(1):182-7.

https://www.ncbi.nlm.nih.gov/pubmed/17228046

4. Kelly A. Meckling, Caitriona O'Sullivan, Dayna Saari. (2004). Comparison of a Low-Fat Diet to a Low-Carbohydrate Diet on Weight Loss, Body Composition, and Risk Factors for Diabetes and Cardiovascular Disease in Free-Living, Overweight Men and Women. 2004; 89 (6): 2717-2723. doi: 10.1210/jc.2003-031606 https://academic.oup.com/jcem/article-lookup/doi/10.1210/jc.2003-031606

5. William S. Yancy, MD, MHS; Maren K. Olsen, PhD; John R. Guyton, MD; Ronna P. Bakst, RD; Eric C. Westman, MD, MHS. (2004). A Low-Carbohydrate, Ketogenic Diet versus a Low-Fat Diet To Treat Obesity

and Hyperlipidemia: A Randomized, Controlled Trial. Published: Ann Intern Med. 2004;140(10):769-777.

DOI: 10.7326/0003-4819-140-10-200405180-00006 http://annals.org/aim/article/717451/low-carbohydrate-ketogenic-diet-versus-low-fat-diet-t reat-obesity

6. Volek, J., Sharman, M., Gómez, A., Judelson, D., Rubin, M., Watson, G., ... Kraemer, W. (2004). Comparison of energy-restricted very low-carbohydrate and low-fat diets on weight loss and body composition in overweight men and women. Nutrition & Metabolism, 1, 13.   http://doi.org/10.1186/1743-7075-1-13 https://www.ncbi.nlm.nih.gov/pmc/articles/PMC538279/

7. Gasior, M., Rogawski, M. A., & Hartman, A. L. (2006). Neuroprotective and disease-modifying effects of the ketogenic diet. Behavioural Pharmacology, 17(5-6), 431–439.

https://www.ncbi.nlm.nih.gov/pmc/articles/PMC2367001/

8. Bonnie J. Brehm, Randy J. Seeley, Stephen R. Daniels, David A. D'Alessio. (2003). A Randomized Trial Comparing a Very Low Carbohydrate Diet and a Calorie-Restricted Low Fat Diet on Body Weight and Cardiovascular Risk Factors in Healthy Women. 2003; 88 (4): 1617-1623. doi: 10.1210/jc.2002-021480 https://academic.oup.com/jcem/article-lookup/doi/10.1210/jc.2002-021480

9. Hemingway C, Freeman JM, Pillas DJ, Pyzik PL. (2001). The ketogenic diet: a 3- to 6-year follow-up of 150 children enrolled prospectively. Pediatrics. 2001 Oct;108(4):898-905.

https://www.ncbi.nlm.nih.gov/pubmed/11581442

10. Zhou, W., Mukherjee, P., Kiebish, M. A., Markis, W. T., Mantis, J. G., & Seyfried, T. N. (2007). The calorically restricted ketogenic diet, an effective alternative therapy for malignant brain cancer. Nutrition & Metabolism, 4, 5. http://doi.org/10.1186/1743-7075-4-5 https://www.ncbi.nlm.nih.gov/pmc/articles/PMC1819381 /

11.	Daikhin Y, Yudkoff M. (1998). Ketone bodies and brain glutamate and GABA metabolism. Dev Neurosci.	1998;20(4-5):358-64. https://www.ncbi.nlm.nih.gov/pubmed/9778572

12.	Yudkoff M, Daikhin Y, Nissim I, Lazarow A, Nissim I. (2001). Ketogenic diet, amino acid metabolism, and seizure control. J Neurosci Res. 2001 Dec 1;66(5):931-40. https://www.ncbi.nlm.nih.gov/pubmed

13.	Website article: Emily Deans M.D. (2011). Your Brain on Ketones – How a high-fat diet can help the brain work better.

https://www.psychologytoday.com/blog/evolutionary-psychiatry/201104/your-brain-keton es

14.	Yudkoff M, Daikhin Y, Melø TM, Nissim I, Sonnewald U, Nissim I. (2007). The ketogenic diet and brain metabolism of amino acids: relationship to the anticonvulsant effect. Annu Rev Nutr. 2007;27:415-30. https://www.ncbi.nlm.nih.gov/pubmed/17444813

15.	Erecińska M, Nelson D, Daikhin Y, Yudkoff M. (1996). Regulation of GABA level in rat brain synaptosomes: fluxes through enzymes of the GABA shunt and effects of glutamate, calcium, and ketone bodies. J Neurochem. 1996 Dec;67(6):2325-34. https://www.ncbi.nlm.nih.gov/pubmed/8931464/

16.	Wang ZJ, Bergqvist C, Hunter JV, Jin D, Wang DJ, Wehrli S, Zimmerman RA. (2003). In vivo measurement of brain metabolites using two-dimensional double-quantum MR

spectroscopy--exploration of GABA levels in a ketogenic diet. Magn Reson Med. 2003 Apr;49(4):615-9.

https://www.ncbi.nlm.nih.gov/pubmed/12652530/

17.	Phinney, S. D. (2004). Ketogenic diets and physical performance. Nutrition & Metabolism, 1, 2. http://doi.org/10.1186/1743-7075-1-2

https://www.ncbi.nlm.nih.gov/pmc/articles/PMC524027/

Choosing the right magnesium supplement for you can be confusing. That's why we share these guidelines with you.

The Bad Forms of Magnesium

- Magnesium oxide

o Only 4% absorbed (https://www.ncbi.nlm.nih.gov/pubmed/11794633)

o Will not help with anxiety

o Not effective in increasing overall magnesium levels

o Laxative

- Magnesium sulfate

o Generally too harsh for oral use

o Laxative (can cause serious diarrhea)

o 32 official FDA reports of magnesium sulfate triggering brain fog, short-term memory loss, amnesia, and other kinds of mental distress. (http://www.druginformer.com/search/side_effect_details /magnesium%20sulfate/ amnesia.html)

- Magnesium glutamate & aspartate

○ Glutamic acid and aspartic acid are components of the dangerous artificial sweetener aspartame, and both of them become neurotoxic when not bound to other amino acids.

The Good Forms of Magnesium

- Magnesium citrate

○ Easily absorbed (https://www.ncbi.nlm.nih.gov/pubmed/14596323)

○ Mild constipation aid

- Magnesium taurate

○ Easily absorbed

○ Calming effects

○ Helps with heart arrhythmia and high blood pressure

● Magnesium malate

○ Easily absorbed

○ Prevents fatigue

(https://www.ncbi.nlm.nih.gov/pubmed/20109177)

○ Effective in treating fibromyalgia (https://www.ncbi.nlm.nih.gov/pubmed/8587088) (https://www.researchgate.net/publication/232047086_M anagement_of_Fibromy algia_Rationale_for_the_Use_of_Magnesium_and_Malic _Acid)

● Magnesium glycinate

o Very easily absorbed, and thus ideal for treating deficiency

o Calming effect

• Magnesium chloride

o Detoxes cells and tissues (http://drsircus.com/medicine/magnesium/magnesium-chloride-benefits)

o Can boost metabolism

• Magnesium carbonate

o Easily absorbed

o Turns into magnesium chloride in the stomach

o Has antacid properties

Magnesium l-threonate, the only form of magnesium that can enter the brain?

Magnesium l-threonate is a little known source of magnesium that might be particularly helpful for the brain. It is the only form of magnesium known to permeate the blood brain barrier.

(https://www.sciencedaily.com/releases/2010/02/10022 2162011.htm)

(https://www.ncbi.nlm.nih.gov/pubmed/20152124)

Results from animal studies have indicated that magnesium l-threonate might be effective in treating anxiety and depression.

(https://www.ncbi.nlm.nih.gov/pmc/articles/PMC393678
3/)

There are no results from human studies yet. And l-threonate is not the best for treating a magnesium deficiency due to its relatively low content of elemental magnesium per dose.

Magnesium Dosage

The recommended daily allowance of (elemental) magnesium for adults is generally 430mg for men and 320mg for women.

(https://ods.od.nih.gov/factsheets/Magnesium-HealthProfessional/)

Many people benefit from even higher doses.

Some recommend starting with 700 mg to kickstart your magnesium into the normal range

(http://drcarolyndean.com/2012/10/when-magnesium-makes-me-worse/)

"Hands down, bar none and without a doubt, the top supplement for anxiety is magnesium and in my experience, if it doesn't work that means you haven't taken enough."

—Dr. Carolyn Dean

(http://drcarolyndean.com/2014/06/is-anxiety-a-magnesium-deficiency/)

It can be a good idea to get magnesium in several different forms.

The Quality of Your Supplement

LabDoor.com has analyzed supplements at independent research facilities and tested them for purity, safety, label accuracy, nutritional value, and projected efficacy.

Here is their list ranking different magnesium supplements:

https://labdoor.com/rankings/magnesium

Further reading:

http://bebrainfit.com/choose-nutritional-supplements/

http://bebrainfit.com/magnesium-anxiety-stress/

http://www.naturalnews.com/046401_magnesium_diet

ary_supplements_nutrient_absorption.ht

ml

http://examine.com/supplements/Magnesium/

Disclaimer

We do not advocate nutritional supplementation over proper medical advice or treatment. This course is not intended to provide diagnosis, treatment or medical advice. Please consult with a physician or other healthcare professional regarding any medical or health related diagnosis or treatment options.

Choosing the right zinc supplement can be confusing. That's why we share these guidelines.

Good forms of zinc supplements include zinc picolinate, zinc gluconate, zinc acetate, and zinc citrate, with studies indicating that zinc picolinate has the best absorption. [1]

Zinc salts such as zinc sulfate (ZnSO) and zinc oxide (ZnO) are not easily absorbed by the

4

body, and should be avoided in supplements.

Zinc Dosage

The Reference Daily Intake, or Recommended Daily Intake (RDI), is the daily intake level of a nutrient that is

Zinc Requirements Daily Reference Intakes

Infants		Males	
0 - 6 months	2 Zinc(mg/day)	9 - 13 years	8 Zinc(mg/day)
7 - 12 months	3 Zinc(mg/day)	14 - 18 years	11 Zinc(mg/day)
		19 - 30 years	11 Zinc(mg/day)
Children		31 - 50 years	11 Zinc(mg/day)
1 - 3 years	3 Zinc(mg/day)	51 - 70 years	11 Zinc(mg/day)
4 - 8 years	5 Zinc(mg/day)	> 70 years	11 Zinc(mg/day)
Pregnancy		Females	
< 18 years	13 Zinc(mg/day)	9 - 13 years	8 Zinc(mg/day)
19 - 30 years	11 Zinc(mg/day)	14 - 18 years	9 Zinc(mg/day)
31 - 50 years	11 Zinc(mg/day)	19 - 30 years	8 Zinc(mg/day)
		31 - 50 years	8 Zinc(mg/day)
Lactation		51 - 70 years	8 Zinc(mg/day)
< 18 years	14 Zinc(mg/day)	> 70 years	8 Zinc(mg/day)
19 - 30 years	12 Zinc(mg/day)		
31 - 50 years	12 Zinc(mg/day)		

considered to be sufficient to meet the requirements of 97–98% of healthy individuals in every demographic in the United States.

Fig. 1:Zinc Requirements Daily Reference Intakes. [2]

The optimal nutrition level is in general higher than the RDI numbers, sometimes much higher, but we do not know what those numbers are. Furthermore, individual optimal nutrition levels vary with age, sex, health status and genetic makeup. [2]

The optimal dosage is probably somewhere between the reference daily intake seen in fig. 1 and the Tolerable Upper Limit of Intake (TUL) of 40mg. [3]

A zinc intake much higher than the TUL over long periods of time might promote health issues such as decreased immune function, copper deficiency, and gastrointestinal effects. [4]

The Quality of Your Supplement

LabDoor.com has analyzed supplements at independent research facilities and tested them for purity, safety, label accuracy, nutritional value, and projected efficacy.

Here is their list ranking different zinc supplements:

https://labdoor.com/rankings/zinc

Further reading:

Dietary factors influencing zinc absorption:

http://jn.nutrition.org/content/130/5/1378S.full

A potential medicinal importance of zinc in human health and chronic disease:

https://www.researchgate.net/profile/Debjit_Bhowmik4/p

ublication/277014212_A_potential_med

icinal_importance_of_zinc_in_human_health_and_chron

ic_disease/links/555ec6ea08ae86c06b 5f4d7f.pdf

Zinc and its importance for human health: An integrative review:

https://www.ncbi.nlm.nih.gov/pmc/articles/PMC3724 376/

References:

[1]   Barrie SA, Wright JV, Pizzorno JE, Kutter E, Barron PC. (1987) Comparative absorption of zinc picolinate, zinc citrate and zinc gluconate in humans. https://www.ncbi.nlm.nih.gov/pubmed/3630857

[2]   Debjit Bhowmik, Chiranjib, K.P. Sampath Kumar. (2010) A potential medicinal importance of zinc in human health and chronic disease. https://www.researchgate.net/profile/Debjit_Bhowmik4/publication/277014212_A_potential_med icinal_importance_of_zinc_in_human_health_and_chron ic_disease/links/555ec6ea08ae86c06b 5f4d7f.pdf

[3]   Fact sheet found here:

https://examine.com/supplements/zinc/

[4]   Laura M. Plum, Lothar Rink, and Hajo Haase. (2010) The Essential Toxin: Impact of Zinc on Human Health.

https://www.ncbi.nlm.nih.gov/pmc/articles/PMC2872 358/